GIANNA DANIELS

Healthy Eating/Healthy Living

40 Dish Recipes For Diabetic Patients

Dedicated to God and family

Contents

Acknowledgement

Acknowledge the contribution of my colleagues most especially Mrs Chioma.

INTRODUCTION

Successfully managing diabetes requires a long-term commitment to healthy eating habits and lifestyle changes. One key aspect of diabetes management is being aware of one's carbohydrate and sugar intake. This means choosing foods that are nutritious and keeping portions in check to help regulate blood sugar levels. Fortunately, there are many delicious and healthy meal options that can help diabetics maintain their health.

To simplify the process of meal planning, we have compiled a list of 40 nutritious meals specifically designed for people with diabetes. These meals are not only healthy but also delicious, making it easier to stick to a diabetes-friendly diet without feeling deprived.

By incorporating these meals into your diet, you can enjoy a wide variety of foods while keeping your blood sugar levels under control. With a little planning and preparation, you can successfully manage your diabetes and maintain a healthy lifestyle for years to come.

Brussels Sprouts

russels sprouts are a nutritious and versatile vegetable that offer several health benefits. Here are some potential benefits of Brussels sprouts and a recipe to try:

Health Benefits:

1. High in Fiber: Brussels sprouts are a good source of dietary fiber, which can help regulate digestion, lower cholesterol levels, and reduce the risk of chronic diseases such as heart disease and diabetes.

2. Vitamins and Minerals: Brussels sprouts are a good source of vitamin C, vitamin K, vitamin A, folate, and other nutrients that support overall health, including immune function, bone health, and blood pressure regulation.

3. Antioxidants: Brussels sprouts are rich in antioxidants, which can help protect against cellular damage and reduce the risk of chronic diseases such as cancer and Alzheimer's disease.

4. Anti-inflammatory: Brussels sprouts contain compounds that have anti-inflammatory properties, which can help reduce inflammation in the body and support overall health.

Recipe:

Here's a simple and delicious recipe for roasted Brussels sprouts with garlic and lemon:

Ingredients:
- 1 pound Brussels sprouts, trimmed and halved
- 2 cloves garlic, minced
- 2 tablespoons olive oil
- Salt and pepper, to taste
- Juice of 1/2 lemon

Instructions:

1. Preheat the oven to 400°F.

2. In a large bowl, toss the Brussels sprouts with the garlic, olive oil, salt, and pepper.

3. Transfer the Brussels sprouts to a baking sheet and roast for 20-25 minutes, or until tender and lightly browned.

4. Remove the Brussels sprouts from the oven and drizzle with lemon juice.

5. Serve and enjoy!

This recipe can be customized by adding other herbs or spices, such as rosemary or paprika, or by topping with grated parmesan cheese or toasted nuts.

Turkey breast with whole-grain mustard

Turkey breast with whole-grain mustard is a flavorful and healthy dish that provides several potential health benefits. Here are some of the benefits and a recipe to try:

Health Benefits:

1. Lean Protein: Turkey breast is a lean source of protein that can help support muscle growth and repair, as well as provide a feeling of fullness to aid in weight management.

2. Whole-Grain Mustard: Mustard is a good source of vitamins and minerals, including vitamin C, calcium, and iron. Whole-grain mustard can provide additional fiber and antioxidants to support overall health.

3. Low in Fat: Turkey breast with whole-grain mustard is a low-fat meal option that can be a healthy addition to any diet.

Recipe:

Here's a simple recipe for turkey breast with whole-grain mustard:

Ingredients:
- 1 pound turkey breast
- 2 tablespoons whole-grain mustard
- 2 cloves garlic, minced
- 1 tablespoon olive oil
- Salt and pepper, to taste

Instructions:

1. Preheat the oven to 375°F.

2. In a small bowl, mix together the whole-grain mustard, minced garlic, olive oil, salt, and pepper.

3. Rub the mustard mixture all over the turkey breast, making sure it is evenly coated.

4. Place the turkey breast in a baking dish and roast in the oven for 30-40 minutes, or until the internal temperature reaches 165°F.

5. Let the turkey breast rest for a few minutes before slicing and serving.

This recipe can be customized by adding other seasonings or herbs, such as thyme or rosemary, or by using different types of mustard. Turkey breast with whole-grain mustard can be served with a side of vegetables or a grain, such as quinoa or brown rice, for a balanced meal.

Spinach Omelet

Spinach omelets are a healthy and delicious breakfast option that offer several potential health benefits. Here are some of the benefits and a recipe to try:

Health Benefits:

1. High in Protein: Eggs are a good source of high-quality protein, which can help support muscle growth, repair, and maintenance.

2. Vitamins and Minerals: Spinach is a good source of vitamins A, C, and K, as well as minerals such as iron and calcium. These nutrients can help support overall health, including immune function, bone health, and blood pressure regulation.

3. Low in Carbs: Spinach omelets are a good option for those following a low-carb or keto diet.

4. Antioxidants: Spinach contains antioxidants such as beta-carotene and lutein, which can help protect against cellular damage and reduce the risk of chronic diseases such as cancer and heart disease.

Recipe:

Here's a simple recipe for a spinach omelet:

Ingredients:
  - 2 large eggs
  - 1/2 cup fresh spinach leaves
  - 1/4 cup shredded cheese (optional)
  - Salt and pepper, to taste
  - 1 tablespoon olive oil or butter

Instructions:

1. In a small bowl, beat the eggs with a fork or whisk until well blended. Season with salt and pepper to taste.

2. Heat the olive oil or butter in a non-stick skillet over medium heat.

3. Add the spinach leaves to the skillet and cook for 1-2 minutes, or until wilted.

4. Pour the beaten eggs into the skillet and cook for 2-3 minutes, or until the edges are set.

5. Sprinkle the cheese over half of the omelet, if using.

6. Using a spatula, fold the other half of the omelet over the cheese and cook for an additional 1-2 minutes, or until the cheese is melted and the eggs are cooked through.

7. Slide the omelet onto a plate and serve hot.

This recipe can be customized by adding other vegetables or herbs, such as mushrooms or thyme, or by using a different type of cheese.

8

Garlic Roasted Cauliflower

Garlic roasted cauliflower is a delicious and nutritious dish that can provide several potential health benefits. Here are some of the benefits and a recipe to try:

Health Benefits:

1. High in Nutrients: Cauliflower is a good source of vitamins C and K, folate, and fiber. These nutrients can help support overall health, including immune function, bone health, and digestion.

2. Antioxidants: Cauliflower contains antioxidants such as beta-carotene and vitamin C, which can help protect against cellular damage and reduce the risk of chronic diseases such as cancer and heart disease.

3. Anti-Inflammatory: Cauliflower contains compounds that have anti-inflammatory properties, which can help reduce inflammation in the body and support overall health.

4. Low in Calories: Cauliflower is a low-calorie vegetable that can be a healthy addition to any diet.

Recipe:

Here's a simple recipe for garlic roasted cauliflower:

Ingredients:
- 1 head cauliflower, cut into florets
- 2 tablespoons olive oil
- 3 cloves garlic, minced
- 1/2 teaspoon salt
- 1/4 teaspoon black pepper

Instructions:

1. Preheat the oven to 425°F.

2. In a large bowl, toss the cauliflower florets with the olive oil, minced garlic, salt, and black pepper.

3. Spread the cauliflower florets in a single layer on a baking sheet.

4. Roast the cauliflower in the oven for 20-25 minutes, or until it is tender and lightly browned.

5. Remove the cauliflower from the oven and let it cool for a few minutes.

6. Serve the garlic roasted cauliflower hot and enjoy!

This recipe can be customized by adding other seasonings, such as paprika or cumin, or by adding other vegetables, such as onions or carrots. Garlic roasted cauliflower can also be used as a side dish or as a base for other dishes, such as cauliflower fried rice or cauliflower pizza crust.

Zucchini Noodles

Zucchini noodles, also known as zoodles, are a popular low-carb and gluten-free alternative to traditional pasta. Here are some of the potential health benefits of zucchini noodles and a recipe to try:

Health Benefits:

1. Low in Calories: Zucchini noodles are very low in calories, which can help with weight loss and weight management.

2. High in Fiber: Zucchini noodles are a good source of dietary fiber, which can help regulate digestion, lower cholesterol levels, and reduce the risk of chronic diseases such as heart disease and diabetes.

3. Vitamins and Minerals: Zucchini is a good source of vitamin C, vitamin A, potassium, and other nutrients that support overall health, including immune function, bone health, and blood pressure regulation.

4. Low in Carbs: Zucchini noodles are a good alternative to traditional pasta for those following a low-carb or keto diet.

Recipe:

Here's a simple recipe for zucchini noodles with garlic and parmesan:

Ingredients:
- 3 medium zucchinis, spiralized
- 2 cloves garlic, minced
- 2 tablespoons olive oil
- Salt and pepper, to taste
- 1/4 cup grated parmesan cheese
- Optional toppings: chopped parsley, red pepper flakes

Instructions:

1. Heat the olive oil in a large skillet over medium heat.

2. Add the garlic and sauté for 1-2 minutes, or until fragrant.

3. Add the zucchini noodles to the skillet and toss to coat in the garlic oil. Cook for 2-3 minutes, or until the noodles are tender.

4. Season with salt and pepper to taste.

5. Remove the skillet from the heat and sprinkle with parmesan cheese.

6. Top with chopped parsley and red pepper flakes, if desired.

7. Serve and enjoy!

This recipe is easy to customize by adding your favorite protein or vegetables, such as grilled chicken or cherry tomatoes.

Spinach Soup

S pinach soup is a delicious and nutritious dish that can provide several potential health benefits. Here are some of the benefits and a recipe to try:

Health Benefits:

1. Rich in Nutrients: Spinach is a good source of vitamins A, C, and K, as well as minerals such as iron and calcium. These nutrients can help support overall health, including immune function, bone health, and blood pressure regulation.

2. Anti-Inflammatory: Spinach contains compounds that have anti-inflammatory properties, which can help reduce inflammation in the body and support overall health.

3. Digestive Health: Spinach is high in fiber, which can help regulate digestion and promote bowel regularity.

4. Antioxidants: Spinach contains antioxidants such as beta-carotene and lutein, which can help protect against cellular damage and reduce the risk of chronic diseases such as cancer and heart disease.

Recipe:

Here's a simple recipe for spinach soup:

Ingredients:
- 1 tablespoon olive oil
- 1 medium onion, chopped
- 2 cloves garlic, minced
- 4 cups vegetable broth
- 2 cups packed fresh spinach leaves
- Salt and pepper, to taste
- 1/4 cup heavy cream (optional)

Instructions:

1. In a large pot, heat the olive oil over medium heat.

2. Add the chopped onion and garlic to the pot and sauté for 2-3 minutes, or until softened.

3. Add the vegetable broth to the pot and bring to a simmer.

4. Add the spinach leaves to the pot and stir to combine.

5. Allow the soup to simmer for 5-7 minutes, or until the spinach is wilted and tender.

6. Remove the pot from the heat and let the soup cool slightly.

7. Using an immersion blender, puree the soup until smooth.

8. Season the soup with salt and pepper to taste.

9. Stir in the heavy cream, if using.

10. Serve hot and enjoy!

This recipe can be customized by adding other vegetables or herbs, such as potatoes or thyme, or by using chicken broth instead of vegetable broth.

Turkey Enchiladas

Turkey Enchiladas can offer several health benefits depending on the ingredients used.

Health Benefits:

1. High Protein: Turkey is a good source of lean protein, which is essential for building and repairing tissues in the body. A serving of turkey enchiladas can provide a good amount of protein.
2. Fiber: Whole grain tortillas and black beans, which are often used in turkey enchiladas, are good sources of fiber. Fiber can help regulate digestion, promote feelings of fullness, and support heart health.
3. Vitamins and Minerals: Enchiladas made with fresh vegetables such as tomatoes, onions, peppers, and cilantro can provide vitamins and minerals such as vitamin C, vitamin A, and potassium.
4. Reduced Sodium: By making your own enchilada sauce or using low-sodium canned sauce, you can reduce the amount of sodium in your turkey enchiladas compared to pre-packaged or restaurant versions.

Overall, turkey enchiladas can be a healthy and satisfying meal, especially when prepared with fresh ingredients and served with a side of salad or vegetables.

Recipe:

Ingredients:

- 2 cups cooked, shredded turkey meat
    - 1/2 cup chopped onion
    - 1 clove garlic, minced
    - 1/2 cup chopped fresh cilantro
    - 1 can (15 oz) black beans, rinsed and drained
    - 1 can (15 oz) tomato sauce
    - 2 cups shredded cheddar cheese, divided
    - 1 teaspoon ground cumin
    - 1 teaspoon chili powder
    - 8-10 corn tortillas
    - Salt and pepper, to taste
    - Optional toppings: sour cream, sliced jalapenos, diced tomatoes, sliced avocado

Instructions:

1. Preheat the oven to 350°F.

2. In a large bowl, mix together the shredded turkey meat, chopped onion, minced garlic, chopped cilantro, and black beans.

3. In another bowl, mix together the tomato sauce, 1 cup of shredded cheddar cheese, ground cumin, and chili powder.

4. Spread about 1/4 cup of the tomato sauce mixture on the bottom of a 9 by 13 inch baking dish.

5. Warm the corn tortillas in the microwave or in a dry skillet over medium-

high heat until pliable.

6. Place a heaping spoonful of the turkey mixture on each tortilla, roll it up, and place it seam-side down in the baking dish.

7. Once all of the tortillas are filled and rolled up, pour the remaining tomato sauce mixture over the top of the enchiladas.

8. Sprinkle the remaining shredded cheddar cheese over the top.

9. Bake for 20-25 minutes, or until the cheese is melted and bubbly.

10. Serve hot with desired toppings, such as sour cream, sliced jalapenos, diced tomatoes, or sliced avocado.

Roasted Sweet Potato

Roasted sweet potatoes are a delicious and nutritious dish that can provide several potential health benefits. Here are some of the benefits and a recipe to try:

Health Benefits:

1. High in Fiber: Sweet potatoes are high in fiber, which can help regulate digestion and promote bowel regularity.

2. Vitamins and Minerals: Sweet potatoes are a good source of vitamins A, C, and B6, as well as minerals such as potassium and manganese. These nutrients can help support overall health, including immune function, bone health, and blood pressure regulation.

3. Antioxidants: Sweet potatoes contain antioxidants such as beta-carotene and anthocyanins, which can help protect against cellular damage and reduce the risk of chronic diseases such as cancer and heart disease.

4. Anti-Inflammatory: Sweet potatoes contain compounds that have anti-inflammatory properties, which can help reduce inflammation in the body and support overall health.

Recipe:

Here's a simple recipe for roasted sweet potatoes:

Ingredients:
- 2 medium sweet potatoes, peeled and cut into 1-inch cubes
- 2 tablespoons olive oil
- 1 teaspoon salt
- 1/2 teaspoon black pepper
- 1 teaspoon paprika
- 1/2 teaspoon garlic powder

Instructions:

1. Preheat the oven to 400°F.

2. In a large bowl, combine the sweet potato cubes with the olive oil, salt, pepper, paprika, and garlic powder. Toss until the sweet potatoes are evenly coated.

3. Spread the sweet potato cubes in a single layer on a baking sheet.

4. Roast the sweet potatoes in the oven for 20-25 minutes, or until they are tender and lightly browned.

5. Remove the sweet potatoes from the oven and let them cool for a few minutes.

6. Serve the sweet potatoes hot and enjoy!

This recipe can be customized by adding other seasonings, such as cinnamon or cumin, or by adding other vegetables, such as onions or bell peppers.

Roasted sweet potatoes can also be used as a base for other dishes, such as sweet potato and black bean tacos or sweet potato and kale salad.

21

Avocado Toast

Health Benefits:

Avocado is a nutrient-dense fruit that is rich in healthy fats, fiber, vitamins, and minerals. Some of the health benefits of avocado toast include:

- Healthy fats: Avocado is high in heart-healthy monounsaturated fats, which can help improve cholesterol levels and reduce the risk of heart disease.
- Fiber: Avocado is also high in fiber, which can help promote healthy digestion and regulate blood sugar levels.
- Vitamins and minerals: Avocado is a good source of vitamins C, E, K, and B6, as well as folate, potassium, and magnesium, which are essential for overall health.
- Protein: Adding a poached egg or other protein-rich toppings can help increase the protein content of avocado toast, which can help keep you feeling full and satisfied.

Overall, avocado toast is a delicious and nutritious breakfast or snack option that can provide a variety of health benefits.

Recipe:

Ingredients:

- 2 slices of bread
- 1 ripe avocado
- 1 tablespoon lemon juice
- Salt and pepper, to taste
- Optional toppings: sliced tomatoes, crumbled feta cheese, poached egg, sliced radishes, chopped cilantro

Instructions:

1. Toast the bread to your desired level of crispiness.
2. Cut the avocado in half, remove the pit, and scoop out the flesh into a bowl.
3. Mash the avocado with a fork until it reaches your desired level of smoothness.
4. Add lemon juice, salt, and pepper to taste.
5. Spread the avocado mixture onto the toasted bread.
6. Add any desired toppings, such as sliced tomatoes, crumbled feta cheese, poached egg, sliced radishes, or chopped cilantro.
7. Serve and enjoy!

Quinoa Vegetable Pilaf

Quinoa Vegetable Pilaf is a nutritious and flavorful dish that offers several health benefits.

Health Benefits:

1. High in Fiber: Quinoa is a good source of dietary fiber, which can help regulate digestion, lower cholesterol levels, and reduce the risk of chronic diseases such as heart disease and diabetes.
2. Protein: Quinoa is a complete protein, meaning it contains all nine essential amino acids. This makes it an excellent plant-based protein source for vegetarians and vegans.
3. Vitamins and Minerals: The vegetables used in the pilaf, such as carrots, onions, and bell peppers, are rich in vitamins and minerals such as vitamin C, vitamin A, and potassium. These nutrients support overall health, including immune function, bone health, and blood pressure regulation.
4. Antioxidants: Vegetables are also rich in antioxidants, which can help protect against cellular damage and reduce the risk of chronic diseases such as cancer and Alzheimer's disease.
5. Gluten-free: Quinoa is naturally gluten-free, making it a good alternative to wheat-based grains for those with gluten intolerance or celiac disease.

Overall, Quinoa Vegetable Pilaf is a healthy and delicious dish that can provide a range of nutrients and support overall health and wellness.

Recipe:

Ingredients:

- 1 cup quinoa
- 2 cups water
- 2 tablespoons olive oil
- 1 onion, chopped
- 2 cloves garlic, minced
- 1 red bell pepper, diced
- 1 zucchini, diced
- 1 yellow squash, diced
- 1 teaspoon ground cumin
- 1 teaspoon ground coriander
- 1/2 teaspoon turmeric
- Salt and pepper to taste
- 1/4 cup chopped fresh parsley
- 1/4 cup chopped fresh mint
- Lemon wedges for serving

Instructions:

1. Rinse the quinoa in a fine-mesh strainer under cold water and drain well.
2. In a medium saucepan, combine the quinoa and water. Bring to a boil, reduce the heat to low, cover, and simmer for 15-20 minutes, or until the quinoa is tender and the water has been absorbed.
3. While the quinoa is cooking, heat the olive oil in a large skillet over

medium heat. Add the onion and garlic and sauté for 2-3 minutes, or until the onion is soft.

4. Add the red bell pepper, zucchini, and yellow squash to the skillet and sauté for 5-7 minutes, or until the vegetables are tender.

5. Add the cumin, coriander, turmeric, salt, and pepper to the skillet and stir to combine.

6. When the quinoa is cooked, add it to the skillet with the vegetables and stir to combine.

7. Add the chopped parsley and mint to the skillet and stir to combine.

8. Serve the Quinoa Vegetable Pilaf hot, garnished with lemon wedges.

Cauliflower and cheese omelets

Cauliflower and cheese omelets are a delicious and nutritious dish that can provide several potential health benefits. Here are some of the benefits and a recipe to try:

Health Benefits:

1. High in Nutrients: Cauliflower is a good source of vitamins C and K, folate, and fiber. These nutrients can help support overall health, including immune function, bone health, and digestion.

2. Protein: Eggs are a good source of high-quality protein, which can help promote muscle growth and repair.

3. Calcium: Cheese is a good source of calcium, which can help support bone health.

4. Low in Carbs: Cauliflower is a low-carb vegetable that can be a healthy addition to a low-carb or ketogenic diet.

Recipe:

Here's a simple recipe for cauliflower and cheese omelets:

Ingredients:
   - 1 cup cauliflower florets
   - 2 eggs
   - 1/4 cup shredded cheese
   - 1 tablespoon butter
   - Salt and pepper, to taste

Instructions:

1. Steam the cauliflower florets until they are tender.

2. In a small bowl, whisk the eggs together with the shredded cheese and a pinch of salt and pepper.

3. In a nonstick skillet, melt the butter over medium heat.

4. Add the steamed cauliflower to the skillet and cook for 2-3 minutes, stirring occasionally.

5. Pour the egg and cheese mixture into the skillet, spreading it evenly over the cauliflower.

6. Cook the omelet for 3-4 minutes, or until the eggs are set and the cheese is melted.

7. Fold the omelet in half and serve hot.

This recipe can be customized by adding other vegetables, such as spinach or bell peppers, or by using different types of cheese. Cauliflower and cheese omelets can also be served with a side of fresh fruit or toast for a balanced meal.

Roasted potato wedges with rosemary

Roasted potato wedges with rosemary are a delicious and nutritious dish that can provide several potential health benefits. Here are some of the benefits and a recipe to try:

Health Benefits:

1. High in Nutrients: Potatoes are a good source of vitamins C and B6, potassium, and fiber. These nutrients can help support overall health, including immune function, heart health, and digestion.

2. Antioxidants: Rosemary contains antioxidants such as carnosic acid and rosmarinic acid, which can help protect against cellular damage and reduce the risk of chronic diseases such as cancer and Alzheimer's disease.

3. Anti-Inflammatory: Rosemary contains compounds that have anti-inflammatory properties, which can help reduce inflammation in the body and support overall health.

4. Low in Fat: Roasted potato wedges are a low-fat side dish that can be a healthy addition to any meal.

Recipe:

Here's a simple recipe for roasted potato wedges with rosemary:

Ingredients:
- 4-5 medium potatoes, cut into wedges
- 2 tablespoons olive oil
- 1 tablespoon chopped fresh rosemary
- 1/2 teaspoon salt
- 1/4 teaspoon black pepper

Instructions:

1. Preheat the oven to 425°F.

2. In a large bowl, toss the potato wedges with the olive oil, chopped rosemary, salt, and black pepper.

3. Spread the potato wedges in a single layer on a baking sheet.

4. Roast the potato wedges in the oven for 20-25 minutes, or until they are tender and lightly browned.

5. Remove the potato wedges from the oven and let them cool for a few minutes.

6. Serve the roasted potato wedges with rosemary hot and enjoy!

This recipe can be customized by adding other seasonings, such as garlic or paprika, or by using different types of potatoes, such as sweet potatoes or red potatoes. Roasted potato wedges with rosemary can also be served with a side of vegetables or a protein for a balanced meal.

Grilled fish tacos with avocado

Grilled fish tacos with avocado is a tasty and nutritious dish that provides several potential health benefits. Here are some of the benefits and a recipe to try:

Health Benefits:

1. Omega-3 Fatty Acids: Grilled fish is a good source of omega-3 fatty acids, which can help reduce inflammation and lower the risk of heart disease.

2. Protein: Fish is a lean source of protein that can help support muscle growth and repair.

3. Avocado: Avocado is a nutrient-dense food that provides healthy fats, fiber, and vitamins and minerals, including vitamin C, vitamin K, and potassium.

Recipe:

Here's a simple recipe for grilled fish tacos with avocado:

Ingredients:

- 1 pound white fish (such as cod or tilapia), cut into small pieces
- 2 tablespoons olive oil
- 1 teaspoon chili powder
- 1/2 teaspoon garlic powder
- Salt and pepper, to taste
- 8 corn tortillas
- 1 avocado, sliced
- 1/2 cup diced tomatoes
- 1/4 cup chopped fresh cilantro
- Lime wedges, for serving

Instructions:

1. Preheat the grill to medium-high heat.

2. In a small bowl, mix together the olive oil, chili powder, garlic powder, salt, and pepper.

3. Brush the fish with the spice mixture and place on the grill. Cook for 3-4 minutes on each side, or until cooked through.

4. Warm the tortillas on the grill for a minute or two on each side.

5. To assemble the tacos, place some fish on each tortilla and top with sliced avocado, diced tomatoes, and chopped cilantro. Squeeze a lime wedge over each taco before serving.

This recipe can be customized by adding other toppings, such as shredded cabbage, salsa, or sour cream. Grilled fish tacos with avocado can be served with a side of beans or rice for a complete meal.

Rainbow stir-fry

Rainbow stir-fry is a colorful and healthy dish that is easy to prepare and provides numerous health benefits. Here are some of the benefits and a recipe to try:

Health Benefits:

1. Vegetables: A rainbow stir-fry typically includes a variety of colorful vegetables, which provide a range of vitamins, minerals, and antioxidants. These nutrients can help boost immunity, support digestion, and reduce the risk of chronic diseases.

2. Fiber: Vegetables are also a good source of fiber, which can help regulate blood sugar, lower cholesterol, and support healthy digestion.

3. Protein: A rainbow stir-fry can be made with a variety of protein sources, such as tofu, chicken, or shrimp. Protein is essential for muscle growth and repair, and can help keep you feeling full and satisfied.

Recipe:

Here's a simple recipe for rainbow stir-fry:

Ingredients:
- 1 tablespoon vegetable oil
- 2 cloves garlic, minced
- 1 tablespoon fresh ginger, minced
- 1 red bell pepper, sliced
- 1 yellow bell pepper, sliced
- 1 green bell pepper, sliced
- 1 small head of broccoli, chopped into florets
- 1 small carrot, sliced
- 1/2 cup snow peas
- 1/2 cup sliced mushrooms
- 2 tablespoons soy sauce
- 1 tablespoon honey
- 1 teaspoon cornstarch
- 1/4 cup water
- Salt and pepper, to taste
- Cooked rice, for serving

Instructions:

1. In a large skillet or wok, heat the vegetable oil over medium-high heat.

2. Add the garlic and ginger and stir-fry for 30 seconds.

3. Add the bell peppers, broccoli, carrot, snow peas, and mushrooms to the skillet and stir-fry for 5-7 minutes, or until the vegetables are tender-crisp.

4. In a small bowl, whisk together the soy sauce, honey, cornstarch, water,

salt, and pepper.

5. Pour the sauce over the vegetables and stir to coat. Cook for another 2-3 minutes, or until the sauce has thickened.

6. Serve the rainbow stir-fry over cooked rice.

This recipe can be customized by adding or substituting different vegetables or protein sources. Rainbow stir-fry can be a nutritious and satisfying meal on its own or served as a side dish with grilled meat or fish.

Spanish shrimp and cucumber salad

Spanish shrimp and cucumber salad is a refreshing and flavorful dish that is easy to prepare and provides numerous health benefits. Here are some of the benefits and a recipe to try:

Health Benefits:

1. Shrimp: Shrimp is a low-fat, high-protein seafood that is rich in nutrients such as selenium, vitamin B12, and phosphorus. These nutrients can help support healthy brain function, boost immunity, and promote healthy bones and teeth.

2. Cucumber: Cucumber is a low-calorie vegetable that is high in water content and rich in vitamins and minerals such as vitamin C, vitamin K, and potassium. These nutrients can help hydrate the body, support healthy digestion, and reduce inflammation.

3. Olive oil: Olive oil is a heart-healthy oil that is rich in monounsaturated fats, antioxidants, and anti-inflammatory compounds. These nutrients can help reduce the risk of chronic diseases such as heart disease and cancer.

Recipe:

Here's a simple recipe for Spanish shrimp and cucumber salad:

Ingredients:
- 1 pound large cooked shrimp, peeled and deveined
- 1 large cucumber, peeled and diced
- 1/2 red onion, thinly sliced
- 1/4 cup chopped fresh parsley
- 1/4 cup olive oil
- 2 tablespoons sherry vinegar
- 1 teaspoon Dijon mustard
- Salt and pepper, to taste

Instructions:

1. In a large bowl, combine the shrimp, cucumber, red onion, and parsley.

2. In a small bowl, whisk together the olive oil, sherry vinegar, Dijon mustard, salt, and pepper.

3. Pour the dressing over the shrimp and cucumber mixture and toss to coat.

4. Chill the salad in the refrigerator for at least 30 minutes to allow the flavors to meld together.

5. Serve the Spanish shrimp and cucumber salad as a light lunch or as a side dish with grilled meat or fish.

This recipe can be customized by adding additional vegetables or herbs, such as diced tomatoes or chopped cilantro. Spanish shrimp and cucumber salad is a flavorful and nutritious dish that is perfect for warm weather or as a light and healthy meal option.

Greek salad with feta cheese

Greek salad with feta cheese is a delicious and healthy dish that is packed with fresh vegetables, healthy fats, and protein. Here are some of the health benefits and a recipe to try:

Health Benefits:

1. Fresh vegetables: Greek salad typically includes a variety of fresh vegetables, such as lettuce, tomatoes, cucumbers, onions, and bell peppers. These vegetables are rich in vitamins, minerals, and fiber, which can help support overall health and wellbeing.

2. Feta cheese: Feta cheese is a low-fat cheese that is rich in protein and calcium. Protein is essential for building and repairing muscle tissue, while calcium is important for healthy bones and teeth.

3. Olives: Olives are a good source of healthy fats, particularly monounsaturated fats. These fats can help reduce inflammation and lower the risk of heart disease.

Recipe:

Here's a simple recipe for Greek salad with feta cheese:

Ingredients:
- 2 cups chopped lettuce
- 1 cup chopped tomatoes
- 1 cup chopped cucumbers
- 1/2 cup chopped red onion
- 1/2 cup chopped bell pepper
- 1/4 cup chopped Kalamata olives
- 1/2 cup crumbled feta cheese
- 2 tablespoons olive oil
- 1 tablespoon red wine vinegar
- 1 teaspoon dried oregano
- Salt and pepper, to taste

Instructions:

1. In a large bowl, combine the lettuce, tomatoes, cucumbers, red onion, bell pepper, and Kalamata olives.

2. In a small bowl, whisk together the olive oil, red wine vinegar, dried oregano, salt, and pepper.

3. Pour the dressing over the salad and toss to coat.

4. Sprinkle the crumbled feta cheese over the top of the salad.

5. Serve the Greek salad with feta cheese as a light lunch or as a side dish with grilled meat or fish.

This recipe can be customized by adding additional vegetables or herbs, such as chopped parsley or diced avocado. Greek salad with feta cheese is a delicious and healthy dish that is perfect for summer or as a light and refreshing meal option.

Grilled lamb chops with garlic-herb sauce

Grilled lamb chops with garlic-herb sauce is a delicious and healthy dish that is packed with protein, vitamins, and minerals. Here are some of the health benefits and a recipe to try:

Health Benefits:

1. Protein: Lamb chops are a great source of protein, which is essential for building and repairing muscle tissue.

2. Vitamins and minerals: Lamb chops are rich in vitamins and minerals, including iron, zinc, and vitamin B12. Iron is important for healthy red blood cells, while zinc and vitamin B12 are important for a healthy immune system.

3. Garlic: Garlic is a powerful antioxidant and has been shown to have anti-inflammatory properties, which can help reduce the risk of chronic disease.

Recipe:

Here's a simple recipe for grilled lamb chops with garlic-herb sauce:

Ingredients:
- 8 lamb chops
- 2 cloves garlic, minced
- 2 tablespoons fresh parsley, chopped
- 2 tablespoons fresh rosemary, chopped
- 2 tablespoons fresh thyme, chopped
- 1/4 cup olive oil
- Salt and pepper, to taste

Instructions:

1. In a small bowl, whisk together the garlic, parsley, rosemary, thyme, olive oil, salt, and pepper.

2. Brush the garlic-herb sauce over the lamb chops and let them marinate for at least 30 minutes, or up to 24 hours in the refrigerator.

3. Preheat the grill to medium-high heat.

4. Grill the lamb chops for 3-4 minutes per side for medium-rare, or until they reach your desired level of doneness.

5. Remove the lamb chops from the grill and let them rest for 5 minutes.

6. Serve the grilled lamb chops with additional garlic-herb sauce on top.

This recipe can be customized by using different herbs or adding additional seasonings, such as lemon juice or red pepper flakes. Grilled lamb chops with garlic-herb sauce are a delicious and healthy dish that is perfect for a summer barbecue or as a special dinner option.

Zucchini noodles with pesto

Zucchini noodles with pesto is a healthy and delicious dish that is perfect for a light and refreshing meal. Here are some of the health benefits and a recipe to try:

Health Benefits:

1. Low in Calories: Zucchini noodles are low in calories, making them an excellent choice for those looking to maintain a healthy weight.

2. High in Nutrients: Zucchini is a good source of fiber, vitamin C, and potassium, all of which are important for overall health.

3. Healthy Fats: Pesto is made with olive oil and pine nuts, which are both sources of healthy fats that can help improve heart health.

Recipe:

Here's a simple recipe for zucchini noodles with pesto:

Ingredients:

- 3-4 medium zucchini
- 1/2 cup basil leaves
- 1/4 cup pine nuts
- 2 garlic cloves
- 1/4 cup olive oil
- Salt and pepper, to taste

Instructions:

1. Using a spiralizer or vegetable peeler, make zucchini noodles and set them aside.

2. In a food processor, combine basil, pine nuts, garlic, olive oil, salt, and pepper. Blend until the mixture is smooth.

3. In a large bowl, toss the zucchini noodles with the pesto until they are fully coated.

4. Serve the zucchini noodles immediately, topped with additional pine nuts and grated Parmesan cheese, if desired.

This recipe can be easily customized by adding other vegetables, such as cherry tomatoes or roasted bell peppers, or by using different herbs, such as parsley or cilantro. Zucchini noodles with pesto are a healthy and flavorful way to enjoy a low-carb meal that is packed with nutrients.

Whole-grain spaghetti with squash

Whole-grain spaghetti with squash is a healthy and delicious dish that is perfect for a comforting and nutritious meal. Here are some of the health benefits and a recipe to try:

Health Benefits:

1. High in Fiber: Whole-grain spaghetti is high in fiber, which can help regulate digestion and promote satiety.

2. Rich in Vitamins and Minerals: Squash is a good source of vitamin A, vitamin C, potassium, and fiber, all of which are important for overall health.

3. Low in Fat: This dish is low in fat, making it a great choice for those looking to maintain a healthy weight.

Recipe:

Here's a simple recipe for whole-grain spaghetti with squash:

Ingredients:

- 8 oz. whole-grain spaghetti
- 2 small yellow squash, thinly sliced
- 2 small zucchini, thinly sliced
- 1 onion, chopped
- 2 cloves garlic, minced
- 1/4 cup vegetable broth
- 1/4 cup grated Parmesan cheese
- Salt and pepper, to taste

Instructions:

1. Cook the spaghetti according to package instructions until al dente. Drain and set aside.

2. In a large skillet, sauté the onion and garlic in a bit of olive oil until softened.

3. Add the sliced squash and zucchini to the skillet, and continue cooking until the vegetables are tender.

4. Add the vegetable broth to the skillet, and stir to combine. Season with salt and pepper to taste.

5. Toss the cooked spaghetti with the squash mixture in the skillet.

6. Serve the spaghetti immediately, topped with grated Parmesan cheese.

This recipe can be easily customized by adding other vegetables, such as bell peppers or mushrooms, or by using different herbs, such as thyme or rosemary. Whole-grain spaghetti with squash is a healthy and flavorful way to enjoy a comforting and nutritious meal.

Quinoa and black bean burrito bowls

Quinoa and black bean burrito bowls are a delicious and nutritious meal that is easy to prepare and perfect for a quick lunch or dinner. Here are some of the health benefits and a recipe to try:

Health Benefits:

1. High in Protein: Both quinoa and black beans are excellent sources of plant-based protein, making this dish a great option for vegetarians and vegans.

2. Rich in Fiber: Quinoa and black beans are also high in fiber, which can help regulate digestion and promote feelings of fullness.

3. Packed with Nutrients: This dish is also rich in vitamins and minerals, including iron, magnesium, and folate, which are important for overall health.

Recipe:

Here's a simple recipe for quinoa and black bean burrito bowls:

Ingredients:
- 1 cup quinoa, rinsed and drained
- 1 can black beans, rinsed and drained
- 1 red bell pepper, chopped
- 1/2 red onion, chopped
- 1 avocado, sliced
- 1/4 cup chopped fresh cilantro
- 2 tbsp olive oil
- 2 tbsp lime juice
- Salt and pepper, to taste

Instructions:

1. Cook the quinoa according to package instructions until tender and fluffy.

2. In a large skillet, sauté the red bell pepper and red onion in olive oil until softened.

3. Add the black beans to the skillet, and continue cooking until the beans are heated through.

4. In a small bowl, whisk together the olive oil, lime juice, salt, and pepper to make the dressing.

5. Divide the cooked quinoa among four bowls, and top each bowl with the black bean mixture, sliced avocado, and chopped cilantro.

6. Drizzle the dressing over the burrito bowls, and serve immediately.

This recipe can be easily customized by adding other toppings, such as chopped tomatoes, shredded cheese, or sour cream. Quinoa and black bean burrito bowls are a healthy and delicious way to enjoy a satisfying and nutrient-packed meal.

Rice-based Veggie Bowl

Rice-based veggie bowls are a great way to enjoy a delicious and nutritious meal that is packed with vitamins and minerals. Here are some of the health benefits and a recipe to try:

Health Benefits:

1. High in Fiber: Brown rice, which is often used in rice-based veggie bowls, is an excellent source of fiber, which can help regulate digestion and promote feelings of fullness.

2. Rich in Vitamins and Minerals: Veggie bowls are usually made with a variety of colorful vegetables, such as bell peppers, carrots, and spinach, which are rich in vitamins and minerals that are important for overall health.

3. Low in Fat and Calories: Rice-based veggie bowls are generally low in fat and calories, making them a great option for those looking to maintain a healthy weight.

Recipe:

Here's a simple recipe for a rice-based veggie bowl:

Ingredients:

- 1 cup brown rice
    - 1 can chickpeas, drained and rinsed
    - 1 red bell pepper, chopped
    - 1 medium carrot, sliced
    - 1 cup spinach, chopped
    - 1/4 cup chopped fresh parsley
    - 2 tbsp olive oil
    - 2 tbsp lemon juice
    - Salt and pepper, to taste

Instructions:

1. Cook the brown rice according to package instructions until tender and fluffy.

2. In a large skillet, sauté the chickpeas, red bell pepper, and carrot in olive oil until the vegetables are softened.

3. Add the chopped spinach to the skillet, and continue cooking until the spinach is wilted.

4. In a small bowl, whisk together the olive oil, lemon juice, salt, and pepper to make the dressing.

5. Divide the cooked brown rice among four bowls, and top each bowl with the vegetable mixture.

6. Drizzle the dressing over the veggie bowls, and sprinkle with chopped fresh parsley.

This recipe can be easily customized by adding other vegetables or proteins, such as grilled chicken or tofu. Rice-based veggie bowls are a delicious and nutritious way to enjoy a satisfying and healthy meal.

Chicken hummus wrap

Chicken hummus wraps are a delicious and healthy lunch option that can be easily prepared at home. Here are some of the health benefits and a recipe to try:

Health Benefits:

1. High in Protein: Chicken is a great source of protein, which can help keep you feeling full and satisfied for longer periods of time.

2. Rich in Fiber: Wraps made with whole wheat or other whole grain varieties are a good source of fiber, which can help regulate digestion and promote feelings of fullness.

3. Nutritious: Hummus, which is typically used as a spread in chicken hummus wraps, is made with chickpeas, which are high in protein, fiber, and various vitamins and minerals.

Recipe:

Here's a simple recipe for a chicken hummus wrap:

Ingredients:

- 1 whole wheat wrap
    - 4 oz cooked chicken breast, sliced
    - 2 tbsp hummus
    - 1/4 cup sliced cucumber
    - 1/4 cup sliced red bell pepper
    - 1/4 cup sliced red onion
    - 1/4 cup shredded lettuce
    - Salt and pepper, to taste

Instructions:

1. Lay the whole wheat wrap flat on a plate or cutting board.

2. Spread the hummus evenly over the wrap.

3. Layer the sliced chicken, cucumber, red bell pepper, red onion, and shredded lettuce on top of the hummus.

4. Season with salt and pepper, to taste.

5. Fold the sides of the wrap towards the center, and then roll the wrap up tightly from the bottom.

6. Cut the wrap in half, and serve immediately.

This recipe can be easily customized by adding other vegetables or seasonings to the wrap. Chicken hummus wraps are a tasty and healthy lunch option that can be enjoyed on-the-go or at home.

Portobello mushroom burgers

Portobello mushroom burgers are a delicious and healthy alternative to traditional beef burgers. Here are some of the health benefits and a recipe to try:

Health Benefits:

1. Low in Calories: Portobello mushrooms are low in calories and high in fiber, which can help promote feelings of fullness and aid in weight management.

2. Rich in Nutrients: Portobello mushrooms are a good source of potassium, copper, and various B vitamins, which are important for maintaining healthy blood pressure, nerve function, and energy levels.

3. Meatless Option: Choosing a meatless option like a Portobello mushroom burger can be beneficial for reducing saturated fat and increasing the intake of plant-based nutrients.

Recipe:

Here's a simple recipe for a Portobello mushroom burger:

Ingredients:

- 4 Portobello mushroom caps
    - 1 tbsp olive oil
    - 2 tbsp balsamic vinegar
    - 1 clove garlic, minced
    - 1/2 tsp dried basil
    - Salt and pepper, to taste
    - 4 whole wheat burger buns
    - 4 slices of cheese (optional)
    - Toppings of your choice (lettuce, tomato, onion, avocado, etc.)

Instructions:

1. Preheat the grill or a grill pan to medium-high heat.

2. In a small bowl, whisk together the olive oil, balsamic vinegar, garlic, and dried basil.

3. Remove the stems from the Portobello mushrooms and brush the caps with the olive oil mixture.

4. Season the mushrooms with salt and pepper.

5. Grill the Portobello mushrooms, gill side down, for about 4-5 minutes or until they are tender and lightly charred.

6. Flip the mushrooms over and add a slice of cheese to each if desired.

Continue to grill for an additional 1-2 minutes or until the cheese is melted.

7. Toast the burger buns on the grill for about 1-2 minutes.

8. Assemble the burgers by placing the Portobello mushroom cap on the bottom bun and adding your desired toppings.

9. Place the top bun on the burger and serve immediately.

This recipe can be easily customized by adding different seasonings or toppings to the burger. Portobello mushroom burgers are a tasty and healthy option that can be enjoyed by vegetarians and meat-eaters alike.

Eggplant tomato Parmesan

Eggplant Tomato Parmesan is a delicious and healthy dish that is packed with flavor and nutrients. Here are some of the health benefits and a recipe to try:

Health Benefits:

1. High in Fiber: Eggplant and tomatoes are both high in fiber, which can help keep you feeling full and satisfied for longer periods of time. This can aid in weight management and support digestive health.

2. Rich in Antioxidants: Eggplant and tomatoes are both rich in antioxidants, which can help protect the body against cellular damage and inflammation. This can support overall health and reduce the risk of chronic diseases.

3. Low in Calories: This dish is low in calories and fat, making it a great option for those looking to reduce their calorie intake and support weight loss.

Recipe:

Here's a simple recipe for Eggplant Tomato Parmesan:

Ingredients:

- 2 medium eggplants, sliced into 1/4 inch rounds
    - 2 cups of tomato sauce
    - 1/2 cup of grated Parmesan cheese
    - 1/2 cup of breadcrumbs
    - 1/4 cup of chopped fresh basil
    - 2 cloves of garlic, minced
    - Salt and pepper to taste
    - Olive oil for cooking

Instructions:

1. Preheat the oven to 375°F (190°C).

2. Line a baking sheet with parchment paper and lightly brush the eggplant slices with olive oil on both sides.

3. Place the eggplant slices on the baking sheet and sprinkle them with salt and pepper.

4. Roast the eggplant slices in the preheated oven for about 20-25 minutes or until they are soft and slightly golden.

5. In a small bowl, mix together the Parmesan cheese, breadcrumbs, garlic, and chopped basil.

6. In a 9x13 inch baking dish, spread a thin layer of tomato sauce on the

bottom.

7. Arrange a layer of eggplant slices on top of the tomato sauce.

8. Spoon more tomato sauce over the eggplant and sprinkle a layer of the Parmesan breadcrumb mixture on top.

9. Repeat these layers until you have used up all of the ingredients.

10. Cover the baking dish with foil and bake for 30 minutes.

11. Remove the foil and bake for an additional 10-15 minutes or until the top is golden brown and bubbly.

12. Serve the Eggplant Tomato Parmesan hot and enjoy!

This recipe can be easily modified to suit your taste preferences. You can add extra vegetables such as zucchini, mushrooms or bell peppers to the dish for extra flavor and nutrients. Eggplant Tomato Parmesan is a healthy and delicious meal that is perfect for any occasion.

Baked Salami

Baked salami is a tasty and easy-to-prepare dish that can be enjoyed as a snack, appetizer, or even a main dish. Here's a recipe and some potential health benefits:

Health benefits:

- Salami is a good source of protein and contains several vitamins and minerals, such as B vitamins and zinc.
- However, it is also high in sodium and saturated fat, so it should be consumed in moderation as part of a balanced diet.
- The honey in this recipe adds a touch of sweetness and may have antibacterial and antioxidant properties, while the olive oil provides heart-healthy monounsaturated fats.

Recipe:

Ingredients:
- 1 lb. salami, sliced
- 1/4 cup Dijon mustard
- 1/4 cup honey

- 1 tbsp. red wine vinegar
- 1 tbsp. olive oil
- 1/2 tsp. garlic powder
- Pinch of salt and pepper

Directions:

1. Preheat the oven to 375°F.
2. Arrange the salami slices in a single layer on a baking sheet lined with parchment paper.
3. In a small bowl, whisk together the mustard, honey, red wine vinegar, olive oil, garlic powder, salt, and pepper.
4. Brush the mixture over the salami slices, making sure to cover each one.
5. Bake for 10-12 minutes, or until the edges are crispy and the salami is heated through.
6. Serve warm or at room temperature.

Risotto with vegetables

Risotto with vegetables is a creamy and satisfying dish that's packed with nutrients. Here's a recipe and some potential health benefits:

Health benefits:

- Risotto rice is a good source of complex carbohydrates and fiber, which can help regulate blood sugar levels and promote digestive health.
- Vegetables like mushrooms, red bell pepper, zucchini, and peas provide a wide range of vitamins, minerals, and antioxidants that are important for overall health.
- Olive oil is a heart-healthy fat that may help lower cholesterol levels and reduce the risk of heart disease.
- Parmesan cheese is a good source of calcium and protein, but should be consumed in moderation due to its high sodium content.

Recipe:

Ingredients:
- 1 onion, diced
- 2 cloves garlic, minced

- 1 cup arborio rice
- 4 cups vegetable broth
- 1 cup sliced mushrooms
- 1 red bell pepper, diced
- 1 zucchini, diced
- 1 cup frozen peas
- 1/4 cup grated Parmesan cheese
- 2 tbsp. olive oil
- Salt and pepper to taste
- Chopped fresh herbs for garnish (optional)

Directions:

1. In a large saucepan or Dutch oven, heat the olive oil over medium heat. Add the onion and garlic and sauté until softened, about 3-4 minutes.
2. Add the arborio rice and stir until coated with the oil and slightly toasted, about 2-3 minutes.
3. Add the vegetable broth, one cup at a time, stirring frequently and waiting for the liquid to be absorbed before adding more.
4. After about 20-25 minutes, the rice should be tender and creamy. If the rice is not fully cooked, continue adding broth and stirring until it is.
5. In a separate pan, sauté the mushrooms, red bell pepper, zucchini, and frozen peas until tender.
6. Add the sautéed vegetables to the risotto and stir to combine.
7. Stir in the grated Parmesan cheese and season with salt and pepper to taste.
8. Serve hot, garnished with chopped fresh herbs if desired.

Chili con carne

Chili con carne is a spicy stew that originated in Texas and is now popular all over the world. It is typically made with ground beef, tomatoes, chili peppers, onions, and spices, and is often served with rice or cornbread. Here is a recipe for chili con carne:

Health benefits:

- Protein: Ground beef is a good source of protein, which is important for building and repairing muscles, skin, and other tissues in the body.
- Fiber: The kidney beans and black beans in chili con carne are high in fiber, which can help regulate digestion and promote feelings of fullness.
- Vitamins and minerals: Tomatoes and bell peppers are rich in vitamin C, which is important for immune system function, and potassium, which helps regulate blood pressure. Chili powder contains small amounts of iron and vitamin A.

Recipe:

Ingredients:
- 1 lb ground beef

- 1 onion, chopped
- 1 green bell pepper, chopped
- 3 cloves garlic, minced
- 1 can (14.5 oz) diced tomatoes, undrained
- 1 can (8 oz) tomato sauce
- 1 can (15 oz) kidney beans, drained and rinsed
- 1 can (15 oz) black beans, drained and rinsed
- 1 tbsp chili powder
- 1 tsp cumin
- 1 tsp paprika
- 1/2 tsp oregano
- Salt and pepper, to taste
- Shredded cheese and chopped green onions, for garnish

Instructions:

1. In a large pot or Dutch oven, cook the ground beef over medium heat until browned, breaking it up into small pieces as it cooks.

2. Add the chopped onion, green bell pepper, and garlic to the pot and cook for another 5 minutes, stirring occasionally.

3. Stir in the diced tomatoes, tomato sauce, kidney beans, black beans, chili powder, cumin, paprika, oregano, salt, and pepper.

4. Bring the chili to a simmer and cook for 30-40 minutes, stirring occasionally, until the flavors have melded together and the chili has thickened to your liking.

5. Serve hot, garnished with shredded cheese and chopped green onions, if desired.

Health benefits:

- Protein: Ground beef is a good source of protein, which is important for building and repairing muscles, skin, and other tissues in the body.

- Fiber: The kidney beans and black beans in chili con carne are high in fiber, which can help regulate digestion and promote feelings of fullness.

- Vitamins and minerals: Tomatoes and bell peppers are rich in vitamin C, which is important for immune system function, and potassium, which helps regulate blood pressure. Chili powder contains small amounts of iron and vitamin A.

Tuna stuffed tomatoes

Tuna stuffed tomatoes are a tasty and healthy meal option that can be made quickly and easily. Here is a recipe and some health benefits of this dish:

Health benefits:

1. High in protein: Tuna is a great source of protein, which is essential for building and repairing tissues in the body.
2. Low in calories: Tuna stuffed tomatoes are a low-calorie meal option that can help with weight management.
3. Rich in vitamins and minerals: Tomatoes are packed with nutrients like vitamin C, vitamin K, and potassium, which are important for maintaining good health.

Note: It is important to choose tuna that is sustainably sourced and low in mercury.

Recipe:

Ingredients:
- 4 medium-sized tomatoes
- 1 can of tuna in water, drained
- 2 tablespoons of mayonnaise
- 1 tablespoon of chopped red onion
- 1 tablespoon of chopped fresh parsley
- Salt and pepper to taste

Directions:

1. Cut off the tops of the tomatoes and scoop out the flesh and seeds with a spoon.
2. In a bowl, mix together the tuna, mayonnaise, red onion, and parsley.
3. Season the mixture with salt and pepper to taste.
4. Stuff the tuna mixture into the hollowed-out tomatoes.
5. Place the stuffed tomatoes onto a baking sheet and bake in a preheated oven at 375°F for 15-20 minutes, or until the tomatoes are tender and the tuna mixture is heated through.

Health benefits:

1. High in protein: Tuna is a great source of protein, which is essential for building and repairing tissues in the body.
2. Low in calories: Tuna stuffed tomatoes are a low-calorie meal option that can help with weight management.
3. Rich in vitamins and minerals: Tomatoes are packed with nutrients like vitamin C, vitamin K, and potassium, which are important for maintaining good health.

Note: It is important to choose tuna that is sustainably sourced and low in mercury.

72

Beef and cabbage stir-fry

Here is a recipe for beef and cabbage stir-fry along with some of its health benefits:

Health benefits:

1. Rich in protein: Beef is a great source of protein, which is essential for building and repairing tissues in the body.
2. High in fiber: Cabbage is rich in fiber, which can help promote healthy digestion and prevent constipation.
3. Low in calories: This stir-fry is a low-calorie meal option that can help with weight management.
4. Rich in vitamins and minerals: Cabbage is packed with nutrients like vitamin C, vitamin K, and potassium, which are important for maintaining good health.

Recipe:

Ingredients:
- 1 pound of beef sirloin, thinly sliced
- 1 head of cabbage, thinly sliced
- 2 carrots, peeled and julienned

- 1 red bell pepper, thinly sliced
- 1 onion, thinly sliced
- 2 garlic cloves, minced
- 2 tablespoons of soy sauce
- 1 tablespoon of honey
- 1 tablespoon of sesame oil
- 1 tablespoon of vegetable oil
- Salt and pepper to taste
- Green onions and sesame seeds for garnish

Directions:

1. In a small bowl, whisk together soy sauce, honey, and sesame oil. Set aside.
2. Heat vegetable oil in a large skillet over medium-high heat.
3. Add beef slices and stir-fry for 2-3 minutes until browned. Remove beef from skillet and set aside.
4. In the same skillet, add garlic, onion, carrots, and red bell pepper. Stir-fry for 3-4 minutes until vegetables are slightly softened.
5. Add cabbage to the skillet and stir-fry for an additional 2-3 minutes until cabbage is tender but still slightly crisp.
6. Return beef to the skillet and pour in the soy sauce mixture. Stir-fry for an additional 1-2 minutes until everything is well combined and heated through.
7. Season with salt and pepper to taste.
8. Serve hot, garnished with sliced green onions and sesame seeds.

Health benefits:

1. Rich in protein: Beef is a great source of protein, which is essential for building and repairing tissues in the body.
2. High in fiber: Cabbage is rich in fiber, which can help promote healthy

digestion and prevent constipation.

3. Low in calories: This stir-fry is a low-calorie meal option that can help with weight management.

4. Rich in vitamins and minerals: Cabbage is packed with nutrients like vitamin C, vitamin K, and potassium, which are important for maintaining good health.

Honey garlic salmon

H oney garlic salmon is a delicious and nutritious dish that is easy to prepare. Here's the recipe and health benefits:

Health Benefits:

Salmon is an excellent source of protein, omega-3 fatty acids, and vitamin D. Omega-3 fatty acids are known to reduce inflammation, lower blood pressure, and improve brain function. Additionally, honey is a natural sweetener that provides antioxidants, while garlic is known for its antibacterial properties and ability to boost the immune system. Overall, this dish is a healthy and flavorful way to enjoy the benefits of these nutritious ingredients.

Recipe:

Ingredients:
- 4 salmon fillets
- 3 tbsp honey
- 2 tbsp soy sauce
- 1 tbsp minced garlic
- 1 tbsp rice vinegar

- 1 tbsp olive oil
- Salt and black pepper to taste
- Lemon wedges for serving
- Fresh parsley or cilantro for garnish

Instructions:

1. Preheat the oven to 375°F (190°C).
2. In a small bowl, whisk together the honey, soy sauce, minced garlic, rice vinegar, olive oil, salt, and black pepper.
3. Line a baking dish with foil and place the salmon fillets in it. Brush the honey garlic sauce over the salmon fillets, making sure to coat them evenly.
4. Bake the salmon for 12-15 minutes, or until the flesh is cooked through and flakes easily with a fork.
5. Serve the honey garlic salmon hot, garnished with fresh parsley or cilantro and lemon wedges on the side.

Skillet eggs and spinach

Skillet eggs and spinach is a nutritious and easy-to-make breakfast or brunch dish. Here's the recipe and health benefits:

Health Benefits:

This dish is a great source of protein, healthy fats, and fiber. Spinach is rich in vitamins and minerals, including vitamin A, vitamin C, and iron, which are essential for maintaining healthy skin, hair, and bones. Eggs are a good source of protein and contain vitamins and minerals such as vitamin D, vitamin B12, and selenium. Additionally, olive oil provides healthy monounsaturated fats and is associated with a lower risk of heart disease. Overall, this dish is a nutritious and tasty way to start your day.

Recipe:

Ingredients:
- 4 eggs
- 4 cups fresh spinach leaves
- 1/2 onion, chopped
- 2 garlic cloves, minced

- 1 tbsp olive oil
- Salt and black pepper to taste
- Grated Parmesan cheese for serving

Instructions:

1. In a large skillet, heat the olive oil over medium-high heat. Add the chopped onion and minced garlic and sauté for 2-3 minutes, or until the onion is translucent.
2. Add the fresh spinach leaves to the skillet and stir until they are wilted and tender, about 2-3 minutes.
3. Create four small wells in the spinach mixture and crack an egg into each well.
4. Cover the skillet with a lid and cook the eggs until the whites are set and the yolks are cooked to your desired doneness, about 3-5 minutes.
5. Season the skillet eggs and spinach with salt and black pepper to taste and sprinkle grated Parmesan cheese over the top before serving.

Sweet potato hash

R ecipe for sweet potato hash and its health benefits:

Health benefits:

Sweet potatoes are a great source of vitamins A and C, fiber, and potassium. They also contain antioxidants that may help reduce inflammation in the body. Eggs, which are a key ingredient in this recipe, provide high-quality protein and important vitamins and minerals, including vitamin D and choline.

Recipe:

Ingredients:
- 1 large sweet potato, peeled and diced into small cubes
- 1 small onion, diced
- 1 red bell pepper, diced
- 2 cloves garlic, minced
- 2 tablespoons olive oil
- Salt and pepper to taste
- 4 eggs

Instructions:

1. Heat the olive oil in a large skillet over medium-high heat.
2. Add the diced sweet potato, onion, and red bell pepper to the skillet, and season with salt and pepper.
3. Cook the vegetables for 8-10 minutes, stirring occasionally, until the sweet potatoes are tender and the other vegetables are softened.
4. Add the minced garlic to the skillet, and cook for an additional minute.
5. Push the vegetables to the sides of the skillet to create a well in the center.
6. Crack the eggs into the well, and season them with salt and pepper.
7. Cover the skillet with a lid, and cook the eggs for 3-5 minutes, until the whites are set but the yolks are still runny.
8. Serve the sweet potato hash hot, with the eggs on top.

Enjoy your delicious and healthy sweet potato hash!

Tofu & broccoli stir-fry

Tofu and broccoli stir-fry is a healthy and delicious vegan dish that's easy to prepare. Here's a recipe and the health benefits:

Health benefits:

- Tofu is a good source of protein, and it's also high in iron and calcium.
- Broccoli is low in calories but high in fiber, vitamins, and minerals, such as vitamin C, vitamin K, and potassium.
- Red bell pepper is rich in vitamin C, which is essential for healthy skin, hair, and immune system.
- Onion and garlic contain compounds that have been shown to have anti-inflammatory and antibacterial properties, which may help boost immunity and fight infections.
- Soy sauce is high in sodium, so it should be consumed in moderation. However, it also contains antioxidants and may have heart-protective benefits. Cornstarch is used as a thickener for the sauce, but it's low in calories and has no nutritional value.

Recipe:

Ingredients:
- 1 block of firm tofu
- 1 head of broccoli
- 1 red bell pepper
- 1 onion
- 2 cloves of garlic
- 1 tablespoon of vegetable oil
- 2 tablespoons of soy sauce
- 1 tablespoon of cornstarch
- 1 tablespoon of water
- Salt and pepper to taste

Directions:

1. Drain the tofu and pat it dry with paper towels. Cut it into cubes and set it aside.
2. Cut the broccoli into small florets and steam them for 5 minutes or until tender. Set aside.
3. Cut the red bell pepper and onion into thin strips. Mince the garlic.
4. Heat the vegetable oil in a large skillet over medium-high heat.
5. Add the tofu to the skillet and cook until golden brown on all sides, about 5-7 minutes.
6. Add the bell pepper, onion, and garlic to the skillet and stir-fry for 2-3 minutes until they are soft.
7. In a small bowl, mix together the soy sauce, cornstarch, and water until smooth. Pour the mixture over the tofu and vegetables and stir well.
8. Add the steamed broccoli to the skillet and stir-fry for an additional 1-2 minutes until everything is coated with the sauce.
9. Season with salt and pepper to taste and serve hot.

Roasted Veggies with White Bean and Arugula Salad

Roasted Veggies with White Bean and Arugula Salad is a delicious and healthy dish that is easy to make. It's a perfect meal for vegetarians, and it's packed with nutrients that provide a range of health benefits. Here's the recipe:

Health benefits:

- Sweet potatoes are a great source of vitamin A, which supports eye health and immune function, and fiber, which aids digestion.
  - Red onions are high in antioxidants, which can help protect against chronic diseases.
  - Bell peppers are rich in vitamin C, which supports immune function and skin health.
  - White beans are a great source of protein and fiber, which can help keep you full and aid in digestion.
  - Arugula is packed with vitamins A and K, which support eye and bone health, respectively, and is also a good source of antioxidants.

Overall, this dish is a nutritious and tasty way to get a variety of vitamins and minerals into your diet.

Recipe:

Ingredients:
- 1 large sweet potato, peeled and diced
- 1 large red onion, sliced
- 1 large bell pepper, sliced
- 1 can of white beans, drained and rinsed
- 2 cups of arugula
- 2 tablespoons of olive oil
- 1 tablespoon of balsamic vinegar
- Salt and pepper, to taste

Instructions:

1. Preheat the oven to 400°F (200°C).
2. In a large bowl, toss the diced sweet potato, sliced onion, and sliced bell pepper with 1 tablespoon of olive oil and season with salt and pepper.
3. Transfer the vegetables to a baking sheet and roast in the oven for 20-25 minutes, or until the vegetables are tender and lightly browned.
4. While the vegetables are roasting, in a separate bowl, mix the drained and rinsed white beans with 1 tablespoon of olive oil, 1 tablespoon of balsamic vinegar, and a pinch of salt and pepper.
5. When the vegetables are done roasting, remove them from the oven and let them cool for a few minutes.
6. In a large bowl, combine the roasted vegetables and the white bean mixture. Toss until everything is well combined.
7. Add the arugula to the bowl and toss until everything is evenly mixed.
8. Serve the salad warm or at room temperature.

Quinoa-Stuffed Bell Peppers

Quinoa-Stuffed Bell Peppers are a healthy and delicious way to enjoy a flavorful and filling meal. Here's a recipe and the health benefits of this dish:

Health Benefits:

- Quinoa is a complete protein, which means it contains all nine essential amino acids our body needs.
   - Black beans are a good source of fiber, which promotes digestive health and helps regulate blood sugar levels.
   - Bell peppers are low in calories but high in vitamin C and other antioxidants, which help protect the body from damage caused by harmful free radicals.
   - Tomatoes are a good source of lycopene, an antioxidant that may help protect against certain types of cancer.
   - Olive oil is a healthy source of monounsaturated fats, which have been linked to a lower risk of heart disease.

Recipe:

Ingredients:
  - 4 bell peppers (any color)
  - 1 cup quinoa
  - 1 can black beans, rinsed and drained
  - 1 can diced tomatoes, drained
  - 1 small onion, chopped
  - 2 cloves garlic, minced
  - 1 tablespoon olive oil
  - 1 teaspoon chili powder
  - 1/2 teaspoon cumin
  - Salt and pepper, to taste
  - Shredded cheese, for topping (optional)
  - Fresh cilantro, for garnish (optional)

Instructions:

1. Preheat the oven to 375°F.
2. Cut off the tops of the bell peppers and remove the seeds and membranes.
3. In a large skillet, heat the olive oil over medium heat. Add the onion and garlic and cook until soft and fragrant.
4. Add the quinoa, black beans, diced tomatoes, chili powder, cumin, salt, and pepper. Stir to combine and cook until heated through.
5. Stuff the bell peppers with the quinoa mixture and place them in a baking dish.
6. Cover the baking dish with foil and bake for 30-40 minutes or until the bell peppers are tender.
7. Remove the foil and sprinkle shredded cheese over the bell peppers, if desired. Return to the oven and bake until the cheese is melted and bubbly.
8. Garnish with fresh cilantro, if desired, and serve hot.

Yogurt-Marinated Baked Chicken

Sure! Here is a recipe for Yogurt-Marinated Baked Chicken along with its health benefits:

Health benefits:

Yogurt is a good source of protein, calcium, and probiotics, which promote gut health. Chicken is also a good source of protein and contains essential vitamins and minerals, including vitamin B6 and niacin.

Recipe:

Ingredients:

- 1 cup plain yogurt
  - 2 tbsp olive oil
  - 4 garlic cloves, minced
  - 1 tbsp smoked paprika
  - 1 tbsp ground cumin
  - 1 tsp salt
  - 1/2 tsp black pepper

- 4 bone-in chicken breasts

Directions:

1. In a large bowl, whisk together the yogurt, olive oil, garlic, smoked paprika, cumin, salt, and black pepper.

2. Add the chicken breasts to the bowl and toss to coat them well in the marinade.

3. Cover the bowl with plastic wrap and marinate in the refrigerator for at least 30 minutes, or up to 24 hours.

4. Preheat the oven to 375°F.

5. Remove the chicken breasts from the marinade and place them on a baking sheet.

6. Bake for 35-40 minutes, or until the internal temperature of the chicken reaches 165°F.

7. Let the chicken rest for 5 minutes before serving.

Enjoy your flavorful and healthy Yogurt-Marinated Baked Chicken!

Eggplant and potato tarts

Eggplant and potato tarts are a delicious and healthy vegetarian dish that can be served as a main course or side dish. Here's a recipe and some health benefits of the ingredients:

Health benefits:

- Eggplant is a low-calorie vegetable that's high in fiber, vitamins, and minerals. It's a good source of antioxidants and may help lower cholesterol and improve heart health.
- Potatoes are a good source of complex carbohydrates, fiber, and vitamin C. They also contain potassium, which may help lower blood pressure.
- Olive oil is a healthy fat that's rich in antioxidants and anti-inflammatory compounds. It may help reduce the risk of heart disease and other chronic conditions.
- Walnuts are a good source of protein, healthy fats, and antioxidants. They may help reduce inflammation and improve heart health.

Recipe:

Ingredients:
  - 1 medium eggplant, sliced into rounds
  - 2 medium potatoes, peeled and sliced into rounds
  - 1/4 cup olive oil
  - 1/2 teaspoon salt
  - 1/4 teaspoon black pepper
  - 1 tablespoon chopped fresh thyme
  - 1/4 cup grated Parmesan cheese
  - 1/4 cup breadcrumbs
  - 1/4 cup chopped fresh parsley
  - 1/4 cup chopped walnuts (optional)

Instructions:

1. Preheat the oven to 375°F (190°C).
2. In a large bowl, toss the eggplant and potato slices with the olive oil, salt, pepper, and thyme.
3. Arrange the slices in a single layer on a baking sheet.
4. Roast the vegetables for 20-25 minutes, or until they are tender and lightly browned.
5. In a small bowl, combine the Parmesan cheese, breadcrumbs, parsley, and walnuts (if using).
6. Spray a muffin tin with cooking spray.
7. Layer the roasted eggplant and potato slices in the muffin cups, overlapping them to form a shell.
8. Sprinkle the Parmesan breadcrumb mixture on top of each tart.
9. Bake the tarts for 15-20 minutes, or until they are golden brown.
10. Allow the tarts to cool for a few minutes before removing them from the muffin tin and serving.

Vegetable Fried Rice

Vegetable fried rice is a popular and nutritious dish that is easy to make and can be customized to suit your preferences. Here's a recipe for vegetable fried rice along with some health benefits:

Health Benefits:

- Vegetables: This dish is loaded with vegetables, which provide important vitamins, minerals, and fiber. The mix of colorful vegetables adds variety to your diet and provides a range of health benefits.
  - Brown rice: Using brown rice instead of white rice increases the fiber and nutrient content of the dish. Brown rice is a good source of magnesium, phosphorus, and B vitamins.
  - Eggs: Eggs are a good source of protein, vitamins, and minerals. They also contain antioxidants that can protect your eyes from damage.
  - Soy sauce: Soy sauce is a good source of umami flavor and adds depth to the dish. It also contains antioxidants and can help lower blood pressure.

Recipe:

Ingredients:
  - 2 cups cooked rice (preferably leftover)
  - 2 tablespoons oil
  - 1 small onion, diced
  - 2 cloves garlic, minced
  - 1 teaspoon ginger, minced
  - 1 cup mixed vegetables (such as carrots, peas, bell peppers, broccoli, and corn)
  - 2 eggs, lightly beaten
  - 2 tablespoons soy sauce
  - Salt and pepper, to taste
  - Green onions, chopped (for garnish)

Instructions:

1. Heat the oil in a large skillet over medium-high heat.
2. Add the onion, garlic, and ginger and sauté until fragrant.
3. Add the mixed vegetables and stir-fry for 2-3 minutes, until tender.
4. Push the vegetables to one side of the pan and add the beaten eggs to the other side. Scramble the eggs until fully cooked.
5. Add the cooked rice to the skillet and stir everything together.
6. Add soy sauce, salt, and pepper to taste. Stir well.
7. Continue to cook for 2-3 minutes, stirring occasionally, until everything is heated through.
8. Garnish with chopped green onions.

Quinoa-Mushroom Salad

Sure, here's a recipe for Quinoa-Mushroom Salad:

Health benefits:

- Quinoa is a good source of protein, fiber, and various vitamins and minerals.
  - Mushrooms are low in calories and fat, but high in fiber, vitamins, and antioxidants.
  - Red onions are rich in antioxidants and have anti-inflammatory properties.
  - Parsley and cilantro are both rich in vitamin K and other nutrients.
  - Lemon juice is a good source of vitamin C and antioxidants.

Overall, this quinoa-mushroom salad is a nutrient-dense and delicious option for a healthy meal.

Recipe:

Ingredients:
  - 1 cup quinoa
  - 2 cups water
  - 1/4 teaspoon salt

- 1 tablespoon olive oil
- 1/2 cup sliced mushrooms
- 1/4 cup chopped red onion
- 1/4 cup chopped fresh parsley
- 1/4 cup chopped fresh cilantro
- 2 tablespoons lemon juice
- Salt and black pepper to taste

Instructions:

1. Rinse quinoa in a fine mesh strainer and drain.
2. In a medium saucepan, bring water and 1/4 teaspoon salt to a boil.
3. Add quinoa, reduce heat to low, and simmer for 15-20 minutes or until water is absorbed and quinoa is tender.
4. In a large skillet, heat olive oil over medium-high heat.
5. Add mushrooms and onion and sauté for 5-7 minutes or until mushrooms are tender and lightly browned.
6. In a large bowl, combine cooked quinoa, sautéed mushrooms and onion, parsley, cilantro, and lemon juice.
7. Toss gently to combine.
8. Season with salt and black pepper to taste.
9. Serve chilled or at room temperature.

Baked Salmon with Dill Sauce

Baked salmon with dill sauce is a delicious and healthy recipe that is quick and easy to prepare. Here are the health benefits and recipe:

Health benefits:

Salmon is an excellent source of omega-3 fatty acids, which are essential for heart health and brain function. It is also high in protein, vitamins, and minerals. Dill is a good source of vitamin A and has anti-inflammatory properties.

Recipe:

Ingredients:
- 4 salmon fillets
- 1 tbsp olive oil
- 1 tsp salt
- 1 tsp black pepper
- 2 tbsp fresh dill, chopped
- 1/4 cup plain Greek yogurt
- 1 tbsp lemon juice

- 1 clove garlic, minced

Instructions:

1. Preheat the oven to 400°F (200°C).
2. Place the salmon fillets on a baking sheet and drizzle with olive oil.
3. Season with salt and pepper.
4. Bake for 15-20 minutes, or until the salmon is cooked through.
5. In a small bowl, mix together the dill, Greek yogurt, lemon juice, and garlic.
6. Serve the salmon with the dill sauce on top.

Enjoy your delicious and healthy baked salmon with dill sauce!

About the Author

GIANNA DANIELS is a writer of several amazing cook books